INTERMITTENT FASTING FOR WOMEN OVER 50

The Easy Guide to the Fasting Lifestyle After 50. Take the Gentle Path to Slow Aging, Self Cleansing, Detox Your Body and Support Hormones with Joy and Ease

ELLEN BERRY

Table of Contents

Introduction

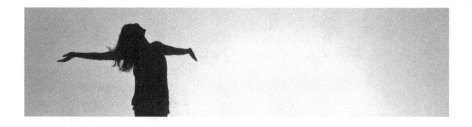

My least favourite thing about intermittent fasting is its name. I know, it's pretty accurate, it tells it like it is, and it is a lot better than the more scientific "metabolic autophagy" that sounds to me like some horror movie from the eighties.

The fact is that the word fasting, however intermittent, recalls in some way sufferance, sacrifice, scarcity, even punishment ("to bed without supper!"), while, in fact, this is the *Exact Opposite*!

If you decide to give intermittent fasting a try, you will discover a lifestyle that is made out of joy, not sufferance, enjoyment, not sacrifice, reward, not punishment. As from the book subtitle "**with joy and ease**".

Intermittent fasting can fit almost everybody, with just a few exceptions, but this book is especially dedicated to women around, and after, the age of 50. While the general information that can be found in this book can benefit almost everyone, there is a reason behind the choice of especially focusing on women over 50 and how intermittent fasting can particularly work for them. Women around that age, nowadays, are often in a phase of their lives when they want to change something for the better.

Maybe you are a successful woman, with an outstanding marriage, a brilliant career, and wonderful kids, and now you are looking at your life realizing that, no matter how wonderful were all your achievements, this may be the first time since your thirties that you can do something just for you. Your job is now stable, the kids heading off to college, you took care of everything and everyone for the last 20, 30 years, now you can (and want, and deserve) take care of yourself.

Or maybe, on the exact opposite, you are not that successful, your life is a mess, you feel like you haven't accomplished anything. And you feel that you are still young, but not as young as 20 years ago, and the moment to stop wasting your energies and start focusing on yourself has come.

Now, chances are that you are neither the completely fulfilled Mrs Perfect of case one nor the miserable wreck of case two. You are more likely, just like the most of us, somewhere in between. You have had your highs and lows, victories and defeats, peaks and valleys. Be that as it may, you may be now in that place where you want to take care of yourself, enjoy your present moment, cultivate a better you, starting from your everyday habits

Habits. Yes, that's what I like the most about intermittent fasting: it is not what you eat, it is how, and when, you do it. You don't have to wonder all the time "can I eat this? Can I eat that? How much can I have of this? How many times a week?".

Intermittent fasting is not exactly a diet. It is more of an eating plan that can fit into our lives, and does not make each meal an exercise of counting and calculating calories and nutrients. While it isn't for everybody, people who are not satisfied with their present dietary patterns might be keen on the health benefits of eating less regular meals and in a potential increment in your body's capacity to process the nutrients you take in.

People on an intermittent fasting plan, for the most part, refrain from eating during the fasting time frame yet get a few calories as low-calorie refreshments, for example, espresso or tea.

It may sound somewhat outrageous to propose fasting every day for sixteen hours and eating for just eight hours. However, in practice, you are fasting for six to eight hours consistently every night, if you are getting the generally prescribed amount of rest. That is up to half of your fasting time if you are following a 16/8 Intermittent Fasting plan, which most likely makes the possibility of a sixteen-hour fast considerably less overwhelming.

Following an intermittent fasting plan does not imply cutting calories or nutrients, but instead that you get the entirety of your nutrients during the eating period. Being in a fasting state will neither make you lose bulk, nor will it weaken your capacity to fabricate new muscles. You can even train in a fasting state.

Intermittent fasting is based on the theory that the sum of food that you take in is less important than the time frames in which you have it.

We are told over and over that ensuring your body a constant supply of protein and amino acids is the ideal approach to a most effective ability to build up muscles. As a matter of facts, it seems there is proof this can hinder your body from building muscle as effectively as possible.

The idea that a consistent source of protein is expected to keep your body in an anabolic state is flawed. Eating high-protein meals a few hours separated is probably not going to activate new muscle development because the amino acid levels in your body do not drain as fast as your protein levels do. Essentially, your body becomes desensitized, over the long term, to elevated levels of protein. Meals more parted can recondition your body's responsiveness to protein and amino acids.

The reduction in muscle protein blend is only one reason why the six meals a day program is flawed. Another imperfection is the effect that frequent meals have on your body's capacity to consume fat, which is a significant one for bodybuilders and for people whose goal is to get slender. Providing your body with a consistent inventory of energy supply implies that it will not have to consume fat.

The six meals a day program is based partially on the idea that you will feel less hungry between meals, making you more reluctant to gorge each time you do eat and less inclined to nibble on unhealthy foods between meals. Nevertheless, this can likewise fail much of the time.

People who get one high-protein meal instead of five littler meals generally feel less craving later on and eat less at their next meal. This frequent meals advice may make you bound to consume extra calories, which is something opposing to the expected effect of diminishing your hunger.

Besides the conceivably negative effect on your body, and the outcomes you get from working out, eating six meals daily can get annoying. Halting what you are doing each a few hours to set up a meal does not typically fit into the daily schedule of most people. Numerous people on a diet dedicate one whole day every week – for the most part toward the end of the week – to set up all of their meals for the upcoming week. Not only would this be able to take up a whole Sunday, yet you would have to purchase, manage, and wash lots of plastic or glass food to bring your meals with you.

There are no hard standards about how to plan your fasting periods. There are basic rules that people largely follow when beginning an intermittent fasting program. Actually, perhaps one of the best points of this type of plan is that it is flexible. You can change your eating timetable to accommodate your way of life as opposed to organizing your whole day around your meals. This means, if one fasting/encouraging schedule does not match your daily routine, you will easily find a way to adjust it.

The vast majority of people on an intermittent fasting plan utilizes a 16/8 plan, which means sixteen hours fasting and eight hours eating. This is commonly the most straightforward calendar to begin with, since around half of your fasting time is during rest, time when you would fast anyway. The eating period will be generally among early afternoon and 8 pm, but as has been said you can adjust it to your needs and habits.

Adapting Intermittent Fasting to Your Everyday Life

One of the most troublesome deterrents to overcome when you initially start intermittent fasting is how your body got used to anticipating frequent meals. Your body's creation of ghrelin, the hormone that makes you feel hunger, adjusts to your general habits. This implies you need to permit it to acclimate to fewer meals, which can take some time.

Following your calorie and macronutrient intake can facilitate the change from your six-meal schedule to an intermittent fasting plan. In case you have been on some kind of diet for any period, you are probably not new to recording what you eat, or monitoring it with some computer software or smartphone application. This will help you with changing over your six little meals into a couple of bigger ones to accommodate your intermittent fasting way of life.

Intermittent fasting is very much adjustable to any calendar, which is probably one of the main reasons why it has such a wide success. Vast numbers of the people who change to an intermittent fasting plan get excited about what a relief it is not to need to invest such a lot of energy preparing and eating food. Since you will never need to worry about food that much, feel free to be flexible, every now and then.

You may have a family occasion involving eating eventually during your fasting period. Some part of the appeal of intermittent fasting is that you never again need to structure your life to suit your dietary patterns, so do not worry about eating when you ought to fast on these casual events.

Chapter 1.

What Intermittent Fasting Is

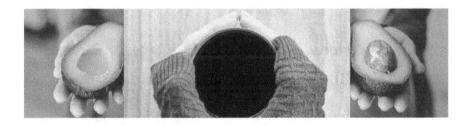

The term intermittent fasting can apply to a number of very different dietary conventions. In contrast to genuine fasting, where no calories are taken during a certain timeframe, intermittent fasting usually allows a few calories even on "fast" days, and those days are distributed among regular calorie "feed" days.

Alternate Day Fasting (ADF)

Alternate day fasting includes intake from zero to 25 percent of every day calorie needs on fasting days, with ordinary intake on regular days. The 5:2 Intermittent Fasting diet is similar, then again, 25 percent of calories are taken on two non-continuous "fast" days during the week, benefiting from the other five days.

Time-Restricted Feeding (TRF)

Time-restricted feeding is not actually fasting in any way, however ordinary eating is restricted to a generally brief timeframe (between 10 am and 6 p.m., for instance), on an ongoing basis.

The most common intermittent fasting methods include alternate days fasting, day-by-day 16-hour fasting, or 24 hours fasting two days per week. For the purpose of this book, the term intermittent fasting will be utilized to portray all of those regimens.

In contrast to most diets, with intermittent fasting is not imposed to keep track of calories or macronutrients. Indeed, there are no recommendations about what foods to eat or avoid, making it even more a way of life than a diet.

Many people utilize intermittent fasting to shed pounds, as it is a basic, advantageous, and successful approach to eat less and diminish body fat.

It might likewise help decrease the danger of heart illness and diabetes, protect bulk, and improve mental clarity.

Additionally, this dietary regime can help spare time in the kitchen as you have fewer meals to plan, prepare, and cook.

Intermittent fasting is an eating plan where you cycle between times of eating and fasting.

It does not utter a word about which foods to eat, yet rather about when you ought to eat them.

There are different types of intermittent fasting methods, all of which split the day or week into eating periods and fasting periods. It is an extremely well known health and wellness pattern, with research to back it up.

Most people already "fast" continuously, while they sleep. Intermittent fasting can be as simple as broadening that fast somewhat more.

You can do this simply by skipping breakfast, eating your first meal around early afternoon and your last meal at 8 pm.

At that point, you are actually fasting for 16 hours consistently and restricting your eating time frame to an 8-hour window. This is the most common type of intermittent fasting, known as the 16/8 plan or method.

In spite of what you may think, intermittent fasting is absolutely simple to follow. Many people report feeling good and having more energy during a fast.

Yearning is generally not unreasonably enormous of an issue, in spite of the fact that it very well may be an issue at the outset, while your body is becoming accustomed to not eating for expanded time frames.

No food is permitted during the fasting period, yet you can drink water, espresso, tea, and other non-caloric refreshments.

A few types of intermittent fasting permit modest quantities of low-calorie foods during the fasting period.

Taking supplements is for the most part permitted while fasting, as long as there are no calories in them.

Benefits of Intermittent Fasting for Women over 50

The general benefits that commonly draw women towards taking up intermittent fasting include:

- Muscle building enhanced and slender

- Increase in energy

- Weight loss

- Increased cell stress response

- Reduced oxidative pressure stress

- Improvement in insulin effectiveness

- Enhanced intellectual capacity

The most significant and immediate benefit you get with the intermittent fasting is weight loss. Other benefits include cell healing, improved emotional wellness, and diminished insulin resistance.

Going back for a moment to the weight-loss effect, here is how it works:

- The intake of standard meals under a shorter time span leaves you feeling satisfied for the entire day.
- During the course of fasting, the body goes into the fasted state. This state cultivates fat consuming, which was not active in the fed state.
- The body goes into the fasted stage in around 8-12 hours after the last meal you take.

This is the motivation behind why you can lose fat without changing the kind and amount of food you eat and the regularity of your workouts.

So let's go a little deeper in the intermittent fasting benefits.

1. *Weight Loss*

The most well known, and looked for, advantage of intermittent fasting is weight loss. Which is understandable, this may also be the main reason why you yourself approached it in the first place. Yet, you may want to explore the topic since there are a lot more advantages that you may not be acquainted with.

As we get older, our digestion system slows down, approaches to perimenopause or menopause and more fat begins accumulating in areas where we do not need it, and intermittent fasting can help.

Some overweight adults who followed an alternate day intermittent fasting plan lost as much as 13 pounds over about two months. Be cautious in case you may want to attempt this strategy in the beginning, since it has some risks such as, for example, eating too much on the days in which you are not fasting.

Not only does intermittent fasting promote fat loss, you likewise hold muscle bulk while fasting, unlike at all typical diets based on calorie cutting.

Intermittent fasting may promote weight loss through a few ways.

To start with, limiting your meals and snacks to a specific time window may for itself diminish your calorie intake, which can help weight loss.

Intermittent fasting may likewise expand levels of norepinephrine, a hormone and neurotransmitter that can help your digestion to increase calorie consuming for the duration of the day.

Moreover, this eating regime may lessen levels of insulin; a hormone associated with glucose. Diminished levels of insulin can knock up fat consumption and increase weight loss.

Some studies even show that intermittent fasting can enable your body to hold bulk more adequately than calorie limitation, which may expand its appeal. Intermittent fasting may diminish body weight by up to 8% and decline body fat by up to 16% over 3–12 weeks.

2. Defective Cells Cleaning

Intermittent fasting promotes autophagy, which is how the body disposes of cells that are more likely to get contaminated or being destructive. Faulty cells not performing at the highest level can accelerate aging, Alzheimer disease, and type 2 diabetes.

The spontaneous repairing procedure happens to go full speed ahead as the body does not need to concentrate on food assimilation. It can completely focus on cell repair. This procedure is called autophagy.

Consequently, fasting helps immediately relieve the body and makes it work properly.

This disposal of "broken" cells is like a spring-cleaning for your body. It makes room for healthy cells and expands your health and dynamic quality.

Fasting makes our cells become stronger regardless of weight loss.

Intermittent Fasting May Have Anti-Aging Benefits

Over the time, researchers have been looking at the conceivable health benefits of calorie limitation for a considerable length of time.

A likely hypothesis suggests these health benefits are due to the drop in glucose that results from fasting, which pushes our cells to work more diligently to use different sources of energy.

Some rhesus monkeys feeded with only 70% of their ordinary caloric intake have appeared to live longer and shown to be healthier in advanced age. This enemy of aging has also been found in animals that were put on an intermittent fasting diet, shifting back and forth between long periods of typical eating and days where calories were restricted.

What is not clear, however, is the reason why intermittent fasting seems to have an important role in the battle against aging. This matter is muddled by the way most of the studies were done on people, when fasting prompted weight loss. The health benefits of weight loss may be overshadowing other benefits acquired from fasting alone.

One way that our cells can be harmed is when they experience oxidative stress. In addition, forestalling or repairing cell damage from oxidative stress is useful in preventing aging. This stress happens when a higher-than-typical generation of free radicals is present.

These stressed particles convey exceptionally receptive electrons.

At the point when one of these free radicals meets another particle, it might either give away or acquire an electron. This can bring about a fast chain response from particle to atom, generating even more free radicals, which can break separated associations between iotas inside significant segments of the cell, like the cell membrane, fundamental proteins, or even DNA. Enemies of oxidants work by moving the required electrons to balance out the free radicals before they can do any harm.

In spite of the fact that fasting appears to enable our cells to fight harm from this procedure, it is not precisely clear how that occurs.

Free radicals can be created by inadequately working mitochondria (the powerhouses of the cell). The switch between eating regularly and fasting makes cells briefly experience lower-than-regular levels of glucose, and they are compelled to start utilizing different sources of less promptly accessible energy, like unsaturated fats. This can make the cells turn on endurance procedures to evacuate the unhealthy mitochondria and replace them with healthy ones over time, subsequently lessening the creation of free radicals in the long term.

The cells may react by expanding their levels of oxidants' common enemies to fight against free radicals creation. In addition, albeit free radicals are usually considered dangerous due to their capacity to harm our cells, they may be significant warning signs for our body.

According to another Harvard University study, intermittent fasting can keep our body more youthful, lengthen our life expectancy, and improve our overall health. Some studies have indicated that intermittent fasting offers no benefits over every day dietary limitations. However, the studies have discovered that it is connected to longer life expectancies.

3. Breast Cancer Recurrence Prevention

A more extended time of fasting is a decent technique to decrease bosom malignant growth recurrence. An investigation of bosom malignancy survivors who didn't eat for any event 12 and half hours overnight showed a 36 percent decrease in the danger of their bosom disease returning.

Intermittent fasting can help your body with resisting the advancement of the disease. The moment we fast, blood glucose levels decline, and the body begins to utilize our fat stores. This secures against the improvement of malignancy in a few different ways:

- Being overweight expands the danger of creating a wide range of types of disease, by getting in shape through intermittent fasting, we can decrease our malignant growth risk.

- Fasting triggers a change from development to repair. When our body changes to repair mode (autophagy), any harmed cells or parts of cells are stalled, and their bits reused to make new, well-working cells. This especially influences cells which may turn harmful.

- Fasting can likewise diminish the amount of the hormone Insulin-like Growth Factor 1 (IGF-1), which is considered related to an expanded malignancy hazard. A few people appear to have especially high IGF-1 levels, and it seems to exist an unbalanced number of malignancy patients with high IGF-1 levels

- The decline in blood glucose prevents malignant growth cells from fuel. Malignant cells, for the most part, cannot utilize fats or ketones for fuel, they just utilize glucose, thus, though normal cells can be perfectly fine with fats or ketones, the diseased cells are famished and cannot develop.

4. Lower Risk of Developing Type 2 Diabetes

Type 2 diabetes frequently creates in people over the age of 45. The Centers for Disease Control and Prevention report that more than 30 million Americans have diabetes (around 1 out of 10), and 90%-95% of these have type 2 diabetes.

Type 2 diabetes can create when your cells do not react properly to insulin. Insulin is a hormone secreted in the intestine by the pancreas, which permits cells to assimilate and utilize glucose (sugar) as energy.

In the event that you become insulin resistant, your cells are not open to insulin and cannot process glucose. Sugar at that point develops in your circulatory system, which can be dangerous. Altogether for your body to get the glucose out of the circulation system, it stores it as fat.

Fasting seems to be related to decreases in glucose and upgrades to insulin effectiveness.

Fasting could offer protection against type 2 diabetes by decreasing the fat storage around the pancreas, German specialists have said.

Has recently been discovered that Intermittent Fasting is able to lower HbA1c (glycated hemoglobin) in people with type two diabetes, just as promoting weight loss. Overweight mice conditioned to be at risk of type 2 diabetes showed a gander at the effect that confining meals at specific times had on fat in the pancreas.

Aggregations outside the fat tissue, for example in liver, muscles, or even bones, negatively affect these organs and the whole body.

5. Boosted and Increased Brain Health

Fasting can soothe cerebrum irritation. Irritation is related to neurological conditions, for example, Alzheimer's disease, Parkinson's disease, and stroke.

Many fasting related effects such as protein sparing, decrease of irritation, autophagy, and increment of BDNF (Brain-derived neurotrophic factor) creation, advantage our cerebrum. From one viewpoint, they decrease the risk of harm to synapses by, for instance, reducing inflammatory reactions. Then again, they additionally favour an appropriate mind work, by advancing cell repair and adding to the arrangement of new synapses and associations between them, in this way encouraging correspondence inside the cerebrum. BDNF specifically increases this structured procedure, and its shortage right now has been connected to psychological issues during aging, for example, dementia. So intermittent fasting has a neuroprotective effect and along these lines promotes a healthy aging.

6. Improved Heart Health

Fasting can prompt a decrease in pulse, heart rate, cholesterol, and triglycerides in people and animals.

Hard to determine what affects fasting has on your heart health because numerous people who routinely fast frequently do as such for health. Therefore these people, for the most part, tend to not smoke and have a healthy lifestyle, which can diminish heart ailment chance.

In any case, some investigations have shown that people who follow a fasting diet tend to have better heart health over people who do not. This might be because people who routinely fast show restraint over what number of calories they eat and drink, and this conduct may convert into weight control and better eating decisions when they are not fasting.

Fasting and better heart health may likewise be connected by the manner in which your body processes cholesterol and sugar. Ordinary fasting can diminish your low-density lipoprotein, or "bad" cholesterol. It is also believed that fasting may improve the way in which your body processes sugar. This can decrease your danger of putting on weight and help treating diabetes, which are both risk factors for a heart ailment.

7. Self Healing

When you are continually eating, you are not giving your body and your cells the time they need to rest. They need this time to repair themselves, or to dispose of those cells that may get tainted or destructive.

Consider your poor stomach continually working. Give it a rest!

The repair procedure happens to go ahead full speed as the body does not need to concentrate on the absorption of food. Therefore it can completely focus on cell repair. This procedure is called autophagy.

This way, fasting helps with restoring your body and makes it work appropriately.

One significant advantage of Intermittent Fasting is that you can focus on tasks better and finish a significant segment of your assignments while in the fasting state.

Insulin resistance happens when you continually have high glucose levels. This prompts the powerlessness of your body to follow up on the sugar content in the blood and separate it.

The point when you take up intermittent fasting, it encourages you to monitor your glucose level.

This condition is also activated by elements like high blood pressure, sedentary lifestyle, inheritance factors, ill-advised diet, or excessive body weight.

In any case, other than all the benefits, there are other things to consider. First is the fasting stage that causes the creation of leptin and ghrelin – the appetite hormones. Nevertheless, women over 50, after some time needed to get used to intermittent fasting, report feeling less ravenous over the long term.

The second point is that intermittent fasting is not recommended for pregnant women. Also, in case a woman who fasts should neglect to take in enough calories, she may have some fruitfulness issues. In any case, if done correctly, there's no reason to worry. In the wake of losing, some overweight women may even improve their fruitfulness.

Downsides of Intermittent Fasting for Women over 50

One can decide to fast for many different reasons, regardless of whether they concern health, weight loss, budget, or religion. Fasting can go from juice-only fasts to fasts that ban all food and liquid, for example, dry fasting. While fasts could have health benefits, they could likewise be risky. Fasting may have contrary effects in the short and long term and adverse effects for some people, including the ones who need to shed pounds. At last, the effects of cutting off food fluctuate a lot, dependent on the person who is fasting.

Weight Management

Fasting could in some cases hinder weight management, as indicated by some dietitians on MayoClinic.com. After a period of fasting, People may develop some issues with starchier foods, or with more fatty substances. Sugars are the body's main source of fuel. Extraordinary appetite likewise makes you pack on a greater number of calories than are healthy for the body. At last, fasting may switch the planned effects on weight management plan.

Short Time Side Effects of Intermittent Fasting

There are a lot of short time side effects of intermittent fasting. These include migraines, dizziness, discombobulation, exhaustion, low blood pressure, and arrhythmia. People who are fasting may experience a weakened ability to carry out some activities, for example, drive vehicles or operating machinery. Fasting could likewise cause flare-ups of specific conditions, for example, gout or gallstones. Fasting could debilitate the body's ability to retain certain meds or even adjust connections in the body.

The long term Side Effects of intermittent Fasting

Short-term side effects of intermittent fasting may have detrimental effects and implications in the long term too. Not only can fasting harm the immune system, it can likewise adversely affect a significant number of organs, including liver and kidneys. Fasting could meddle with substantial crucial capacity. Keeping away from eating could likewise be conceivably hazardous in people who are somehow weakened, for instance, malignant growth patients. It is even possible for fasting to bring about death when the body's put away energy is completely exhausted.

Dry Fasting

There are numerous methods of fasting; dry fasting - avoiding all liquid and food intake - is especially risky. Dry fasting can rapidly prompt parchedness and death within a matter of days. The American Cancer Society reports the health effect of dry fasting shifts largely, dependent on the individual and setting. Factors like, for example, heat, substantial effort, and weakened health, can make dry fasting deadly in simply a question of hours.

Generally speaking, intermittent fasting has a problematic side as well. One of the most common dangers is getting profoundly fixated on following the intermittent fasting plan correctly. Someone could get inflexible in eating, even every now and again, outside the previously fixed plan. For instance, in the event that you have intended to take the primary meal of the day at 12:00 pm, and you are starving by 11:50 am, you may decide to force yourself to wait those 10 minutes. Such over the top dietary patterns are adverse to one's peace of mind, and do not have any positive influence on your physical health.

Lethargy and Overeating

Another significant example of potentially harmful effects of intermittent fasting is the feeling of a never completely fulfilled hunger. Albeit someone is genuinely full, they may be enticed to eat more. This conduct prompts over-eating, and it may kill the inner motivation behind getting in shape that made you start with intermittent fasting.

Another aspect of this downside of intermittent fasting may be the diminished energy levels during the early hours of the day. This outcomes in an individual attitude apathetic and lethargic during work, and furthermore causes decreased willpower levels which can influence one's capacity to do every day exercises.

Increased Hunger

A common symptom of fasting diets is that they may modify the balance of your hormones. In particular, the decrease in leptin, which makes you feel full, and the increase of cortisol, which can bring about your body being under more stress, and accordingly stop weight loss. A Study on fasting indicated female subjects' leptin diminished by as much as 75%, and their cortisol expanded by as quite a bit of 50% after the fasting time. Expanded cortisol can likewise bring about changes in the menstrual cycle for women.

Hormonal Imbalance

Medium build people, who have less weight to lose, and those with really dynamic ways of life are the ones most likely to be prone to suffer this kind of downside of intermittent fasting . As pointed out, the alteration in hormones can prompt sporadic menstrual cycles for women, diminished testosterone in men. Furthermore instances of sleeping disorder and feelings of anxiety were present in all investigation members of both genders. Overweight people who participate in intermittent fasting are most likely to get benefits and have a higher level of fat loss over the fasting period.

From the models over may clearly be derived that we can't affirm that Intermittent Fasting is acceptable or terrible per se. it is up to your initial conditions, current health, body fat rate. In case you intend to go on an intermittent fasting plan, it should be controlled so that its negative outcomes are as negligible as possible.

The most effective method to Succeed with an Intermittent Fasting Plan

There are a few things you have to remember whether you need to shed pounds with intermittent fasting, here below the main four:

1. **Food quality**: The food you eat is still important. Try to eat whole and simply seasoned foods.

2. **Calories**: Calories, despite everything still count. Try to eat "typically" during the eating periods and not to make up for the calories you missed by fasting.

3. **Consistency**: Just like any other weight loss strategy, you have to stick with it for a long term if you want it to work.

4. **Patience**: It will take as much time as is needed to get used to an intermittent fasting lifestyle. Try to be

consistent with your meal calendar, and it will get simpler.

The greater part of the famous intermittent fasting methods also suggests food quality. This is significant in case you need to lose body fat while keeping muscle.

At the beginning, calorie counting is commonly not required with intermittent fasting. If your weight loss slows down, then, calorie counting can be a useful practice.

With intermittent fasting, you, despite everything, need to eat healthily and keep up a calorie shortage if you need to get in shape.

Defining Specific Measurable Goals

Rather than setting a general goal like "getting more fit", be more specific, focus on basic, feasible objectives that should be possible week by week, like:

- Taking a walk three days per week

- Drink 64 ounces of water per day, every day, this week

- Skip one meal this week

Self-Reward When Reaching Small Targets

Set yourself up for progress by utilizing a prize framework. For example:

- After shedding fifteen pounds, get yourself some new clothes.

- If you meet all your monthly goals, treat yourself a massage

The cash spared by skipping a meal (or two) can pay for your prize! Things that can motivate us are different for every one of us, so make sure to find out what might work best for you, and you will stay focused on reaching all of your goals.

Keeping a Journal

This is quite a game-changer. If you have a very strong will power and you are used to doing medium to long term plans and stick to them, you probably won't need to keep a journal, if not for the pleasure to do it, and unless this already is one of the tools behind your willpower.

Most of us though are not like this. The ability to stick to a plan (dietary or of any other nature) is seldom a talent. More often than you think there are tools and practices involved. When it comes to diets, especially, but not only, if the aim is to lose weight, the number one cause of quitting is the lack of immediate and measurable results. Or at least, this is the reason the quitter, in all honesty, gives. But it really is about this? Well, not exactly. Most of the time, it is not that one does not have results, it is that they have in mind the big final goal, therefore they can't appreciate the small ones during the journey.

If your final goal is to save 10.000 dollars, you won't get excited about your first 10 dollars saved. If your final goal is to lift 200 pounds, you won't get excited about your first 20 pounds lifted. If your final goal is to shed 20 pounds, you won't get excited about your first 10 ounces shed. But the truth is, to save 10.000 dollars, to lift 200 pounds, to shed 20 pounds, you have to start saving 10, lifting 20, shedding just your first ten ounces.

This is the main use of journaling: keeping track day by day of the small victories to celebrate and the small struggles to fight, being able to having everything under control and to love and appreciate the journey, until you won't need to keep track anymore and either will quit doing it or will keep on just for the pleasure of it.

Once you know what to keep track of it is very easy, and pleasant, to do it. Not only it is the chance to track your progress, but it also is something that gives you a moment that is all yours, where you can in some way talk to yourself.

I have published an *Intermittent Fasting Journal* that you could use, but you don't necessarily need it. I just published it because it gathers the indicators I usually suggest to track, and I thought for someone would be nice to have a real journal to fill, with some directions on how to use it, but you can simply be inspired by the pictures and do your own journal yourself.

I have set mine as a "three months challenge" because this is, give or take, the period of time in which you may see yourself as a "beginner" of intermittent fasting. Usually, after three months you are in the zone, you just acquired the intermittent fasting lifestyle as your own and you don't need to journal about it anymore (of course you can, someone does it, but it becomes more of a pleasure than a tool).

But of course, this is not set in stone: you can adapt it to your needs.

Here are just some examples of how it is designed.

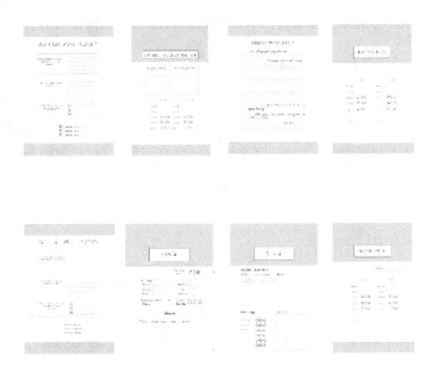

I strongly suggest you keep a journal. If you want you can buy mine (it's called *Intermittent Fasting Journal* and below there is the cover), or you can just look at the pages up here and get inspired to do your own.

Or even, if you want, you can download the pdf version for free here https://forms.aweber.com/form/29/554422929.htm or asking me at zhellenberry@gmail.com then you can print it and use it.

You got so many options, just don't miss the chance of journaling about your intermittent fasting. This will not only help you stay motivated with your new dietary lifestyle, it will also get you used to a tool, journaling, that will be able to help you in countless other situations.

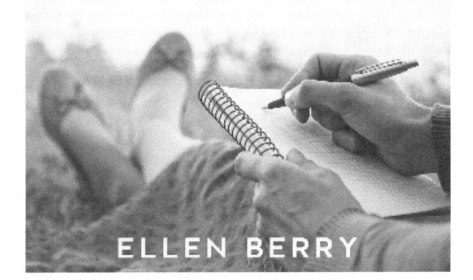

INTERMITTENT FASTING Journal

TRACK YOUR PROGRESS AND ACHIEVEMENTS ON A 90 DAYS
LIFESTYLE JOURNEY, TAKING NOTE OF SMALL AND BIG
IMPROVEMENTS IN YOUR ENERGY, CLARITY AND MOOD

ELLEN BERRY

Chapter 1 Recap

- Intermittent fasting can be divided into two categories: Alternate Day Fasting and Time Restricting Feeding.

- The most famous and immediate benefit of intermittent fasting is weight loss, but there are many others regarding your general body and mind health.

- Weight loss aside, among the main benefits of intermittent fasting we have:
  - Defective cells cleaning
  - Breast cancer recurrence prevention
  - Lower risk of developing type 2 diabetes
  - Boosted and increased brain health
  - Improved heart health
  - Increased self-healing abilities
  - Better focus and mental clarity

- Do not overlook the possible downsides, most of them can be overcome and are usually transitional, nonetheless changing your habits may bring changes to your body, please take care and always check your doctor if something looks wrong.

- Starting with intermittent fasting can seem challenging. Three points can really help you are:
  - Define clear and measurable goals
  - Reward yourself when you get small targets
  - Keep a journal

Chapter 2.

Types of Intermittent Fasting for Women over 50

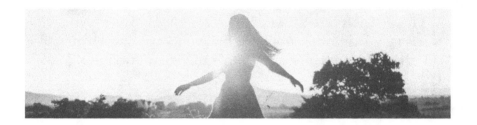

There are countless types of intermittent fasting.

There are so many reasons why decide to follow an intermittent fasting lifestyle, and at least as many methods for doing it. Therefore it is fundamental to set some basic definitions before we go deep in details.

Fasting – giving up the intake of food or anything that has calories for a particular time frame. Normally, some non-caloric beverages and water are allowed.

Intermittent Fasting – to fast intermittently by adding fasts into your regular meal plan.

Extended Fasting – fasting for a drawn-out time span. It will, in general, be cultivated for a significant long time.

Time-Restricted Feeding – restricting your regular food usage inside a particular time window. This is meant to improve the circadian rhythm and general wellness.

Usually, people doing intermittent fasting are restricting their food time and increasing fasting time. To have something like an actual fast, it would need to prop up for over 24 hours, since that is the spot most of the benefits start to kick in.

Now, first let's have an overview on 13 of the main types of intermittent fasting, then we'll go deep in the 6 that better suit women after 50.

1. 24-Hour Fasting

It is the fundamental technique of intermittent fasting – you fast for around 24 hours, and a short time later have a meal. In spite of what the name may suggest, you won't actually go through an entire day without eating. Simply eat around evening, fast all through the next day, and then eat again in the evening.

You can even have your food at the 23-hour check and eat it inside an hour. The idea is to make a very prominent caloric shortage for the day. Most of the benefits will be vain if you, regardless of fasting, binge and put on weight during the eating time frame.

Gradually and occasionally, you can decide to fast according to your physical condition and needs of the moment.

A fit person who works out constantly would require to some degree more eating time frames and less fasting periods.

An overweight person who is sedentary and needs to lose some more weight could follow an intermittent fasting plan as long as they can until they lose the overabundance weight.

2. 16/8 Intermittent Fasting

16:8 intermittent fasting was defined by Martin Berkhan of Leangains. It is used for improving fat loss while not having to go through an extremely demanding process

You fast for 16 hours and eat your food inside 8. What number of meals you have inside that time length is irrelevant, yet whatever it is recommended to keep them around 2-3.

In my opinion, this should be the base fasting length to concentrate on reliably by everybody . There is no physical need to eat any sooner than that and the restriction has many benefits.

A large number of people think that it is more straightforward to postpone breakfast by two or three hours and then eat the last meal around early evening. You should not get insane, and it is demanding to observe the fast. The idea is simply to reduce the proportion of time we spend in an eating state and fast for a large portion of the day.

3. The Warrior Diet

The Warrior Diet is proposed by Ori Hofmekler. He talks about the benefits of fasting on blood pressure through hormesis.

The warrior diet not only improves your body's physical condition and resistance yet, moreover, grows your mental attitude and outlook.

The Warrior Diet talks about old warriors like Spartans and Romans who used to remain on an empty stomach all through the day and eat in the evening. During daylight, they used to stroll around with 40 pounds of armor, build fortresses, and bear the hot sun of the Mediterranean, while having just a quick bite. Around evening time, they would have a huge supper consisting of stews, meat, bread, and many other things.

In the Warrior Diet, you fast for around 20 hours, have a short high power workout, and eat your food during a 4 hours window. Overall, it would merge either two minor meals with a break, or one single huge supper.

4. One Meal a Day OMAD

The One Meal a Day Diet, also called OMAD, simply consists in eating just one big meal every day

With OMAD, you regularly fast around 21-23 hours and eat your food inside a 1-2 hour time slot. This is remarkable for dieting since you can feel full and satisfied once the eating time comes.

It is unmatched for losing fat; be that as it may, not ideal for muscle improvement because of time for protein production and anabolism.

5. 36-Hour Fasting

In the past, people would quite commonly go a couple of days without eating, they probably suffered and yet even thrived. Nowadays, the average person can neither stand to skip breakfast, nor go to bed hungry.

For over 24 hours is the spot where all the magic begins, the more you stay in a fasted state and experience hardship, the more your body is forced to trigger its supply systems that start to draw on fat stores, bolster rejuvenating microorganisms, and reuse old wrecked cell material through the system of autophagy.

It takes, at any rate, an entire day to see major signs of autophagy, yet you can speed it up by eating low carb before starting the fast, rehearsing on an unfilled stomach, and drinking some homemade teas that facilitate the challenge.

For 36 hours is not that irksome truly. You fundamentally eat the night before, don't eat anything during the day, go to sleep on an empty stomach, then wake up the next day, fast a few more hours, and begin eating again.

To make the fasting more straightforward there are, mineral water, plain coffee, green tea, and some homemade teas.

6. 48-Hour Fasting

In case you made it to the 36-hour mark, why not give a try to fast for a straight 48 hours.

It is only irksome getting through the change of habits. Once you overcome this obstacle, which generally occurs around your usual dinnertime, it gets a lot more straightforward.

The moment your body goes into an increasingly significant ketosis phase and autophagy starts, you will overcome hunger, feel very mentally clear, and have greater mindfulness and focus.

The most problematic bit of any complete fast is around the 24-hour mark. If you can make it to fall asleep and wake up the next day, from that moment onward, you have set yourself prepared for fasting for a significant period of time with no issues. You essentially need to get over this hidden obstacle.

Going to bed hungry sounds disturbing; in any case, this is what a huge part of the world's population does daily. This could make you think about your own luck and feel thankful for having food anytime you want.

7. Expanded Fasting (3-7 Days)

48-hours fasting would give you a short ride in autophagy and some fat consuming. To genuinely get the deep health benefits of fasting, you would have to fast for three or more days.

It has been shown that 72-hours of fasting can reset the immune system in mice. Although studies on humans have not confirmed that conclusion, also, there may be some issues in prolonged fastings that are not under severe medical control.

Three to five days is the perfect time frame for autophagy, after which you may begin to see unwanted losses in bulk and muscle. Fasting for seven or more days is not generally suggested. Most people do not need to fast any longer than that since it may make them lose muscle tissue.

Fit people may want to focus on three-four of these expanded fasts every year, to propel cell recovery and clean out the body. Notwithstanding a healthy eating routine without any junk food, I myself do it anyway four times a year because of their tremendous benefits.

In case you are overweight, or you experience the negative effects of some illness, then longer fasts can really help you get back in health. Fast for three to five days, have a little refreshment break, and repeat the plan until needed. I'll never say that enough, if you decide to go through this kind of longer fasting be always sure of what you are doing, and consult a doctor for any doubt.

8. Alternate Day Fasting

Alternate Day Fasting, as for the 5:2 Diet, is a very common type of fasting. Are they fully considered as fasting, nevertheless, despite allowing the intake of 500/660 calories a day on fasting days? Well yes, they are, since these limited amounts of calories are only intended to help extend perseverance.

To have a sporadic caloric intake will not enable the whole of the physiological benefits of fasting to fully manifest. It would limit a part of the effect. In any case, a strict limitation is important for both your physiology and mind.

Everybody can fast. It is just that someone cannot psychologically bear the weight of not to eat. Fasting mimicking diets and alternate day fasting in this respect.

9. *Fasting Mimicking Diet (FMD)*

The Fasting Mimicking Diet, can be used every so often. Commonly, it is followed by people who cannot actually fast like old people or some recovering patients.

Fasting mimicking diet has been shown to reduce blood pressure, lower insulin, and cover IGF-1, all of which have positive benefits on life length. Regardless, these effects are likely an immediate consequence of the huge caloric restriction.

During the Fasting Mimicking Diet, you would eat low protein, moderate carb, and moderate fat foods like mushroom soup, olives, kale wafers, and some nut bars. The idea is to give you something to eat while keeping the calories as low as reasonable. In most cases, again, this is more about satisfying people's psychological needs of eating, than the physical ones.

With zero calories would be just as effective, and it would keep up more muscle tissue by an increasingly significant ketosis.

To thwart unwanted loss of lean mass, you can adapt the macronutrient taken in during Fasting Mimicking Diet and make them more ketogenic by cutting down the carbs and increasing the fats.

10. Protein Sparing Modified Fasting

Protein-Sparing Modified Fast (PSMF) is a low carb, low fat, high protein type of diet that helps getting increasingly fit quite fast, while keeping muscle toned.

Lean mass is a significant matter of stress for healthy people, especially in case they are endeavoring to do intermittent fasting.

A catabolic stressor will, over the long term, lead to muscle loss; notwithstanding, the loss rate is a lot lower than people may imagine. To prevent that from happening, you have to stay in ketosis and lower the body's appetite for glucose.

PSMF is absolutely going to keep up more muscle than the fasting mimicking diet, yet there's the danger of staying out of ketosis in case you are already eating many proteins preparing yourself for muscle catabolism.

11. Fat Fasting

The fasting Physiology and the ketogenic diet may be considered in a general sense equivalent, and both of them start the metabolic state of ketosis.

When you are dieting, i.e. in ketosis, you are using fat and ketones as a basic fuel source instead of glucose. This facilitates you going throughout fasting each day since you will be consuming your own body fat.

Some moderate types of autophagy can safeguard ketones and keep up their effects; nevertheless, it is not as amazing as macro autophagy, which requires the restraint from all calories.

Fat fasting, you can have a pinch of black coffee, 1-2 tablespoons of MCT oil, or some margarine. Anyway anything with carbs or protein in it like bone stock, coconut milk, coconut water, or the like will break the fast.

12. Dry Fasting

Drinking liquids is furthermore said to have autophagic benefits. One-day of dry fasting is thought to ascend to 3 days of water fasting.

The idea is that if you abstain from drinking water, your body will start to change over the triglycerides from the fat tissue into metabolic water. Hydrogen is released because of beta-oxidation.

When in doubt, you should incline toward not to get dehydrated for a truly significant period. Regardless, consistently time-restricted dry fasting of 12-16 hours can be another thing to do if you need further autophagy.

13. Juice Fasting

Do fasting effects show where you just drink juices and smoothies? In reality, it could work likewise of the fasting-mimicking diet.

Vegetables and whole grain products make you intake a genuine basic proportion of starches and fructose, which will all interfere with both ketosis and autophagy exceptionally hard.

You can lose a great deal of weight with juice fasting, yet a huge segment of it will be muscle and fit tissue. This is the reason why you need and should be in ketosis to make the fast effective.

Also, do not use only vegetables like kale or spinach to make a smoothie, you would get in all probability some blockage because of the high proportions of fiber.

If you need to cover hunger or have something to drink that doesn't taste like water, then boil some water with 2 tsp of apple vinegar. It will not stop the fast and truly has uncommon clinical advantages.

Differences Between Types of Intermittent Fasting

The common characteristic is the abstinence from food and drink. The difference, in any case, lies in the point and reason behind fasting, which can go from severe and significant health reasons to shed weight.

A huge amount of what we call 'intermittent fasting' nowadays starts from observational research on Ramadan practices and results.

It is an old practice followed in a large number of countries by masses subject to religion or culture, which by there arrived in the therapeutic world too for healthy reasons.

At now, there is actually inadequate evidence for us to perceive what the ideal number of fasting hours should be to propel results.

Various people consider intermittent fasting as an undeniably versatile dieting strategy that does not require the specific counting of calories, and less overall management

Likewise, it has been shown that intermittent fasting could be as effective for weight loss as any calorie-restricted eating routine.

The 6 Types of Intermittent Fasting to Consider for a Woman over 50

Whether you are just beginning your intermittent fasting path or you have had a go at fasting previously, but you failed to keep it up long term, this guide will help. Discover the seven different types of fasting and which one does better fit to your body, psychology and lifestyle.

There is such a significant number of different approaches to intermittent fasting, that it is impossible to go deep on all of them. In the event that this is something you are keen on doing, you can find the type that will work best for your way of life. Here I selected the most reasonable six:

1. The 5:2 Fasting

It is one of the most well known intermittent fasting methods. Truth be told, the book The Fast Diet made it standard, and structures all that you have to know about this approach. The thought is to eat regularly for five days (with no calorie checks) and afterward the other two eat 500 or 600 calories every day (500 for women, 600 for men), per person. As fasting days you can choose any days based on your personal preference and convenience.

The idea is that short episodes of fasting keep you comfortable. Should you be hungry on a fast day, you simply need to anticipate tomorrow when you can "feast" once more. A few people say 'I can do anything for two days. However, it's a lot to reduce what I eat each of the seven days,'. For these people, a 5:2 approach may win over calorie cutting over the whole week.

All things considered the authors of The Fast Diet advise against making fast days on days where you might be doing a great deal of endurance exercise. In case, you are preparing for a bicycle or running race (or run high-mileage preparation weeks), assess if this kind of fasting could work with your preparation plan or talk with a sport nutritionist.

2. Time-Restricted Feeding

In this type of intermittent fasting, you pick a consistent eating window, which should ideally leave a 14 to 16 hour fast. (Because of hormonal concerns, Women should fast close to 14 hours every day). Fasting advances autophagy, the normal 'cell housecleaning' process where the body clears flotsam and jetsam and other things that hold up the health of mitochondria, which starts when liver glycogen is exhausted.

Doing this may help increase fat cell digestion and enhances insulin work.

To make this work, you may set your eating window from 9 a.m. to 5 p.m., for example. This can work particularly well for somebody with a family, who has an early supper, at any rate. At that point, a significant part of the time invested fasting is spent sleeping in any case. You additionally do not actually need to skip any meals, depending on when you set your window. However, this is subject to how regular your daily schedule can be. In case your timetable is frequently changing, or you need the opportunity to go out for breakfast occasionally, head out for a late-night out in town, or go to party time, day by day times of fasting may not be for you.

3. Overnight Fasting

The method is the least difficult of the bundle and includes fasting for a 12-hour period each day. For instance: Choose to quit having after supper by 7 p.m. furthermore, continue eating at 7 a.m. with breakfast the following morning. Autophagy does, in any case, occur at the 12-hour mark, however, you will get more soft cellular benefits, and this is the base number of fasting hours I would suggest. An upside of this strategy is that it is anything but difficult to actualize. Likewise, you do not need to skip meals; at least, everything you are doing is get rid of your goodnight nibble, if you are used to having one in the first place. This method does not expand the advantages of fasting. In case you are fasting for weight loss, a little fasting window implies more opportunity to eat, and it may not help you with diminishing the number of calories you take in.

4. *Whole Day Fasting*

You eat once every day. A few people decide to have supper and afterward not to eat again until the following day's supper that implies your fasting period is 24 hours. This is different from the 5:2 technique. Fasting periods are 24 hours (supper-to-supper or lunch to lunch), while at 5:2, the fasting is really 36 hours. (For instance, you have supper on Sunday, "fast" Monday by eating 500 to 600 calories, and break it with breakfast on Tuesday.)

An advantage is that, if you are fasting for weight loss, it is very unlikely, if not even impossible, to eat a whole day of calories in just one meal. The downside is that it is difficult to get all the nutrients your body needs to work ideally with only one meal. In addition, this method is hard to follow. You may get extremely ravenous when supper approaches, that can lead you to not ideal nutritional choices, since when you're ravenous you don't usually desire healthy food. Many people also tend to have too much coffee to bear the hunger, which can negatively affect your rest. Some people may likewise experience haze during the day when you are not eating.

5. Alternate Day Fasting

This is the approach proposed by Krista Varady, Phd, nutrition professor at the Illinois University. You can fast every other day, with fasting days consisting of 25 percent of your calorie needs (around 500 calories) and non fasting days being your regular eating days. This is a mainstream approach for weight loss. Alternate day fasting is very effective in helping obese adults losing weight. Side effects like craving diminish after one or two weeks, and you can expect to get used to this regimen and get comfortable after four weeks. The downside is that it may take you the two months or more before you can start feeling really full, which may make this psychologically hard to follow for some people.

6. Pick Your-Day Fasting

You do the time-restricted fasting (fast for 16 hours, eat for eight, for example) each other day or on more days a week. This means, for instance, that Sunday may be a typical day of eating, and you would quit eating by 8 p.m., then at that point, you'd keep eating again on Monday around early afternoon. After all it's like skipping breakfast a couple of days every week.

PYD fasting might be effectively suitable to your lifestyle and is more like taking a path of least resistance, which means you can make it work even with a schedule that changes every week. on the other hand, if you are not very strong willed this could easily lead you to looser methodologies which may mean less powerful benefits.

Chapter 2 Recap

- There are countless types of intermittent fasting. As a woman in her 50s the most reasonable to go for are:

  - The 5:2 Fasting
  - Time-Restricted Feeding
  - Overnight Fasting
  - Whole Day Fasting
  - Alternate Fasting
  - Pick Your Day Fasting

Chapter 3.

What to Eat While Doing Intermittent Fasting

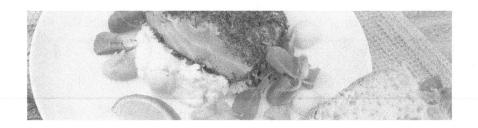

A diet is a way to get more fit and keep up energy levels. Anybody endeavouring to shed pounds should concentrate on nutrients full foods, like fruits, veggies, whole grains, nuts, beans, seeds, just as dairy and high-quality proteins.

High-protein meals can help you to feel full for longer. As protein is usually high in calories, you should not have an excessive amount for your 500 calories. However, try to make protein your fundamental source of calorie.

Full your plate with low-calorie vegetables: they fill your stomach, taste great, and benefit you. Steam them, stew them with a teaspoon of oil, or stir fried with little fat and add a few spices or flavors to make an extremely scrumptious and satiating meal. Also, you can have them crude in a big plate of mixed greens.

Sugars: they are high in calories and make you feel hungry again soon. Examples of starch-containing foods to avoid are potatoes, sweet potato, parsnips, rice, pasta, bread, some fruits (bananas, grapes, melon, prunes, raisins, dates and other dried fruits), breakfast cereal, fruit juice, fresh corn/sweetcorn and anything containing sugar, nectars or syrups.

Fat: don't fear fat. Although fat is high in calories, it makes you feel full. Just remember to have limited fat quantities during your fast day.

And what about instant meals? An instant meal can be an incredibly easy solution. However, as for home-prepared meals, it's advisable to look for low in starch and sugar and high in protein and vegetables alternatives.

At the end of the day, if you follow the following guidelines you will not end up ravenous while fasting.

Water

Since you are not eating, it is critical to remain hydrated for such a huge number of reasons, like the health of essentially every organ. The amount of water that anyone should drink changes, however, you need your pee to be a light yellow. Dark yellow pee shows a lack of hydration, which can cause headaches, weariness, and dizziness. Add this to the food restriction, and you can see how this could be a catastrophe waiting to happen. In case you're not thrilled about the idea of plain water, add a crush of the lemon squeeze, a couple of mint leaves, or cucumber cuts to your water. It will be our little secret.

Avocado

It may look counterintuitive to eat the most fat fruit while trying to get fitter; actually, the avocado's monounsaturated fat is amazingly healthy. Including a portion of an avocado to your lunch may keep you full for quite longer than without eating the "green gold".

Fish

A mainstream dietary guideline suggests eating at any rate eight ounces of fish every week. In addition to the fact that it is rich in protein and healthy fats, it likewise contains plentiful amounts of vitamin D. Moreover, since you are just eating a restricted amount of food during the day, don't you need something that can convey more supplement value for your money? Also, that restricting your calorie intake may upset you a little, and fish is commonly seen as a "brain food"

Cruciferous Vegetables

Broccoli, Brussels sprouts, and cauliflower are, generally, full with fiber. Since you are eating irregularly, it is fundamental to eat fiber-rich foods that will keep you regular and prevent constipation. Fiber also can make you feel full, which is something you may need considering that you won't eat again for 16 hours.

Potatoes

Potatoes are with good reason considered as one of the most satiating foods you can find. Eating potatoes within a balanced and healthy diet could help with weight loss. Curb your enthusiasm ladies, this does not apply to french fries and potato chips.

Beans and Legumes

Legumes may be among your best intermittent fasting friends. Food, especially carbs, supplies energy for staying active. While I am not suggesting you to carbo-load, it wouldn't hurt for sure to put a few low-calorie carbs, like beans and vegetables, into your eating plan. Furthermore, foods like chickpeas, black beans, peas, and lentils have been proved to reduce body weight, even without calorie restriction.

Probiotics

While fasting you may experience some intestine problem due to lack of probiotics, like constipation. To avoid this unpleasant side effect, add probiotic-rich foods to your diet, such as kefir, kombucha, or kraut. The Farmhouse Culture Gut Shots are ideal for any 500-calorie days, since each 1.5 ounce shot is overflowing with live probiotics (10 billion CFUs) for only ten calories.

Berries

Berries are full of crucial nutrients. Strawberries are an incredible source of vitamin C, fundamental for immune system functionality, with more than the whole daily need in just one cup. And in any case, this is not even the best part. Studied on flavonoids have found that people who followed a diet rich in flavonoids, like the ones you can find in blueberries and strawberries, have shown lower increments in BMI, over a many years time span than the people who didn't eat berries.

Eggs

One large egg has six grams of protein and it's ready in minutes. Getting as much protein as possible is fundamental for keeping bulk and building muscle. When you have an egg breakfast rather than a bagel, you will be less hungry and eat less during the day.

Nuts

Nuts might be higher in calories compared to many other snacks, yet nuts contain something that most junk food does not: good fat. Polyunsaturated fat in nuts can really adjust the physiological markers for appetite and satiety.

Moreover, in case you are worried about calories, just relax! A one-ounce serving of almonds (around 20 nuts) gives you 20 percent fewer calories than listed on the label. That's because chewing does not totally transform the almond cells, leaving a part of the nut intact and unabsorbed during digestion.

Whole Grains

Despite a strict eating routine and eating carbs may look like belonging to two different places, that's not entirely true. Whole grains are rich in fiber and protein, so eating a little does his work in keeping you full. Also, eating whole grain rather than refined grains may really speed up your metabolism. So feel free to eat your whole grains and seize the chance to push you out towards foods you may not be used to, such as farro, amaranth, spelled, Kamut, bulgur, millet, freekeh and sorghum.

Chapter 3 Recap

- Intermittent fasting says nothing about what you should or should not eat. Nevertheless, switching to an intermittent fasting lifestyle could be the chance for starting to take care a little more of the quality of what you eat.

- Sugars are high in calories and make you feel hungry again soon.

- Fat is high in calories too, but it makes you feel full, that is good when fasting.

- Food contains water, since you are fasting it is critical that you stay hydrated, so take care to drink more than usual

Chapter 4.

Common Mistakes in Intermittent Fasting

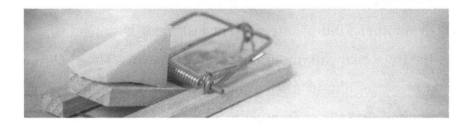

Fasting is not generally seen as a diet, yet a specific way of life and recommended eating schedule. This type of eating plan has increased enormous notoriety as of late, particularly for women over 50. As we have seen, you may fast for 16 hours and eat during an 8-hour window. This is the 16-8 plan and is commonly seen as the standard intermittent fasting plan. A few people follow the alternate day plan, with low calorie intake on one day and the usual amount the following. Whatever the way you handle it, when your goal is to get in shape, intermittent fasting is famous for one peculiar characteristic: it only works when done correctly.

There are a few potential health benefits when following intermittent fasting. Among the benefits we may include decreased danger of malignant growth, diabetes, and heart disease. Fasting can trigger autophagy, which is known to help with dementia. Regardless of whether you utilize one or another kind of intermittent fasting, it is critical to avoid the traps that can undermine your endeavors. Here below are a few intermittent fasting mistakes a lot of people, especially on their first times, frequently make.

Looking for too Many Improvements too Fastly

You are preparing to begin something new, and you are eager to receive all the rewards as fast as could be. It is just normal that you are excited about this new lifestyle and you want to fully dive into it. Nevertheless, attempting to immediately get such a large number of improvements too early may disrupt your endeavors.

The key is to begin gradually by including a couple of changes one after another. For instance, if you have chosen to do two 500 calorie days every week while having a regular amount of calories the other five; consider beginning with only one 500-calorie day. After a couple weeks, you can feel more confident including the second day into your weekly schedule.

Not Taking Care of Your Hydration

Staying in a fasting state can be challenging regardless of whether you are not eating. Most drinks will break the fast and extraordinarily diminish any benefits. Despite the fact that they are fat and calorie free, it is anything but smart to drink "diet" soft drinks. Indeed, even sugars that have zero calories can negatively influence your insulin levels.

The essential fluid you ought to drink during your fast is water. A moderate amount of coffee will not break your fast, but you will need to take your coffee black, in any case. Indeed, even a little sugar in your coffee, like lemon in your water, can influence the fasting period.

Not Drinking Enough Water

While it is crucial not to drink inappropriate fluids when fasting, it is similarly as essential to ensure you drink enough water. Not getting enough water can make you hungry, and it is anything but difficult to sometimes confuse thirst with hunger.

People get a great deal of water from a good part of the foods they eat. Worldwide Food Information states that 20 percent of the water our bodies use originates from food. This implies that in case you are not eating for a few hours you will have to drink around 20 percent more water than usual to compensate for any shortfall.

Eating Unhealthy Foods

Since intermittent fasting is not generally a diet plan, there are not any foods that are "forbidden". This can lead many people to fall into the snare of binge on junk food the moment their fast is up and the eating time opens. Try not to make a habit of unhealthy eating thinking that fasting will compensate for it.

Make a rundown of all the healthy foods you do appreciate. Do ordinary shopping for food and try to stick to your food decisions. While fulfilling your hunger with not exactly healthy snacks sometimes can be all right, for ideal health and weight-loss achievement, it is important to eat as healthy as possible under the circumstances. Eating the right foods is vital to taking advantage of any weight loss plan. Foods rich in calcium, protein, and vitamin B-12 should be high on your grocery list, particularly for women over 50.

Overeating After Each Fast

This is presumably the greatest trap for both beginners and people who have been fasting intermittently for quite a while. Practicing intermittent fasting to get more fit will lose effectiveness if you end up taking in an excessive amount of calories on every chance you have to eat.

One approach to hold back from overeating is to eat larger amounts of healthier foods during your eating window. This would include heaps of healthy plates of mixed greens and crisp vegetables. It is additionally a smart idea to arrange meals and having seasonings prepared before your fast period starts. Thus you are not tempted to just grab anything. Remember that it can take as long as about fourteen days until you have changed and adapted to the point that you will not feel that hungry after each fasting period.

Trying to Stick to the Wrong Plan

There are many different approaches to put intermittent fasting into your daily schedule. For instance, if your fasting plan includes not eating from 8 pm until early afternoon every day and you have a challenging activity that begins right in the first part of the day, this is most likely not the correct plan for you.

What works for one person, may not necessarily fit in for another one. To get the most rewards of intermittent fasting, you should take your time to thoroughly analyze different types of plans. It is all right if it takes a little longer to find out the plan that best works for you.

Working Out Too Much or Too Little

It is critical to remain as dynamic as possible, but you would prefer not to overdo, especially during your fasting times. A few newbies may feel overwhelmed, beginning to follow a new eating schedule, and may overlook exercise altogether. Others might be so enthusiastic that they end up overdoing it.

It is a smart thought to pick a moderate exercise schedule, particularly when beginning. Strolling the pooch for twenty minutes or riding your bicycle to work are simple approaches to add moderate exercise to your customary calendar.

Not Drinking Enough Water

Maybe one of the most common and easily avoidable intermittent fasting mistakes is not taking in enough water.

We know that drinking water is fundamental for overall health, of course, yet it is even more significant when you are fasting.

Why? because most of the time we feel hungry, we are actually dehydrated.

Can you imagine how your hunger might be influenced by lack of water when you are trying to go through the main part of the day without eating?

Fortunately, this is very simple to avoid!

Sneaking more water into your day is as simple as making a couple of basic changes.

A few people truly are bored drinking plain water. Trust me, one thing that may be a great idea is to add a couple of Mio Drops (or other water enhancer) to water. It will have a tremendous effect!

In case you do not know them, Mio Drops are zero-calorie, zero-carb and sugar free water enhancers.

Misunderstanding Real Hunger Signs

Perhaps the best thing that I have learned from my intermittent fasting test is that I found a good pace about when appetite shows.

It does not come at 9 am when I've been awake for one hour and last ate a late-night nibble at 11 pm the prior night.

No doubt, your stomach may be growling, and you may desire for something yummy.

Yet, you are not really hungry.

Also, it may be wonderful to binge with your family or friends and enjoy the social part of feasting.

Yet, again, you are not really hungry.

Intermittent fasting will teach you that if you stand by fasting long enough, more often than not, your "hunger" will blur generally in no more than five or ten minutes.

It most likely already happened without you noticing or giving it a particular thought.

How many times at work you were planning to go to eat, then some however, some last minute rush job showed up, and one hour or two passed by, while you overlooked your stomach's protest?

What before looked like the most urgent priority, eating, was overshadowed by something new that popped up. And you survived!

In any case, yielding and eating too early is one of the serious mix-ups with intermittent fasting. Think that simply drinking some water and allowing it ten minutes or so, you will, usually your appetite will calm down.

Try not to break your intermittent fasting plan before you even begin.

Try not to easily give in to bogus hunger!

Using Intermittent Fasting As an Excuse to Overeat

One of the most harmful intermittent fasting mistakes is give in to the temptation to say, "What the heck, I've starved myself throughout all the day, I deserve to reward myself for supper!", and then diving in a crazy feast of junk food bombing yourself with unhealthy stuff.

Please don't be that woman.

You would feel hopeless, and most likely put on weight.

We don't want that.

In spite of the fact that, actually, intermittent fasting is not a diet because it does not confine what you eat, it is yet critical to settle on healthier food decisions. You want, most of all, to have a healthy relationship with your food and your body.

You can absolutely overeat and put on weight even by eating just once per day, in case you are eating a greater number of calories than your body consumes.

While you do not need to be an absolute stickler and there is space for adaptability, still, be shrewd.

Help yourself out and do not go crazy during your eating window.

Not Eating Enough

If you have yet to attempt intermittent fasting the risk of not eating enough during eating times may appear to be illogical.

Actually, for some people, not eating for a particularly long period of time, it's not unusual to become less hungry.

In some cases, fasting can thoroughly kill your appetite.

Unless you are deliberately doing a total fast (not suggested if not under medical control), however, it is anything but a good idea to decide not to eat enough.

If you should not eat sufficiently for too long, you can easily wreck your digestion and unbalance your hormones.

Moreover, you will deny your body of fundamental nutrients, which can help health avoiding issues that are far more important than the loss of a couple of additional pounds.

Consult your physician about a complete, healthy calorie intake that is fit for weight loss and may help you reach your desired outcomes.

Failing to Plan Your Meals in Advance

While calorie tallying is not important (however truly, you will show more signs of improvement results if you do it), carefully planning and thinking about what you will eat when your eating period arrives is a great intermittent fasting hack.

This will allow you not to have to improvise when you are finally going to sit down at the table.

Rather than going like "I'm starving and need to eat now no matter what" and then heading to the closest, cheapest, and more unhealthy junk food, you better learn to tell yourself "well, I'm feeling hungry now, but I can wait, I'm not dying and something healthy and delicious is waiting for me, later".

Utilizing this opportunity to consider what you will eat when you eat, and sticking to healthier options will only have benefits for you over the long term.

You will learn how to eat for effective weight loss, while decreasing caloric intake, keeping you satisfied, and boosting your self confidence.

In case you are fasting for 16 hours, you can easily invest 5 minutes of your time to plan what meal will break your fast later.

It is really not unreasonably hard and will prepare for a slimmer future!

Not Exercising at All

While it's true that you actually could, in any case, lose a lot of weight with intermittent fasting even without working out at all, why on earth would you pass up the mind-blowing chance to lose significantly more, faster, and with a bunch of other benefits for your health?

It really has neither rhyme nor reason.

Time will be time. A month is a month. In the event that in one month you could be lazy and shed five pounds or exercise three times a week and lose ten, wouldn't you go for the ten?

Chapter 4 Recap

- Regardless of the kind of intermittent fasting it is critical to avoid the most common traps that can undermine your endeavors.

- You are going to start something new and you are full of expectations, that's wonderful, but don't try to get too many improvements in too little time, this would not help your progress but rather may have the opposite effect.

- Don't overeat during your feeding time. Ok, intermittent fasting says nothing about quantities, but don't push it.

- During your fasting you will feel hungry. This is not always real hunger, sometimes it is just the habit of your body to be fed at certains time of the day.

Chapter 5.

Nutritional Facts

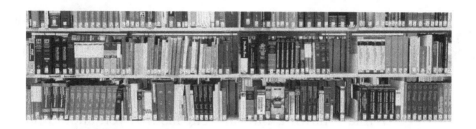

Intermittent fasting is important, yet it is just a hint of something larger about fasting diets overall. There are essentially boundless ways you can embrace a fasting system that suits your own way of life and health needs. We should investigate all the different fasting diets, the health benefits they may bring, and how to do them securely.

As we have seen, intermittent fasting is the voluntary waiving of food for a predefined period, as a rule around 16 hours with a window of 8 hours to expend meals. In most of the cases, this is accomplished by skipping breakfast and having the primary meal of the day at around early afternoon, yet a few people interpret intermittent as meaning restraint of somewhere in the range of 12 to 18 hours.

If you have been following a daily practice of intermittent fasting for quite a while and have been an enthusiastic admirer of this practice, then it is difficult to leave this habit when you are pregnant. Nevertheless, in the event that you are truly bearing a child, you have to change your habits. You have to follow a more regular calendar.

While following intermittent fasting, you should have regularly skipped breakfast and not taken anything after supper. While this can be an incredible way to get thinner, it very well may be a dangerous practice to follow when you are pregnant. Specialists who work in cardiology, weight loss, and eating stress the point that intermittent fasting may play a role in controlling inflammation, cell adjustment, boosting cells repairing, and digestion abilities.

Hormones That Promote Fat Burning

During times of fasting, the body, despite everything, expects energy to work.

This energy can come out of other sources, for example, glycogen (put away glucose) from the muscle and liver, or it can come out of fat.

The moment you fast, and blood glucose drops low, this powers the emission of a hormone from the pancreas called glucagon.

The moment when glucagon levels rise, this starts a process called gluconeogenesis in which the body exchanges over glucose from non-starchy sources, for example, protein, or discharges glucose from the liver.

On the other hand, this glucagon expansion can start a procedure of using fat for energy, one of the principle benefits of intermittent fasting.

Strikingly, fasting likewise expands levels of hormones called catecholamines.

These catecholamine hormones can join to receptors situated on the films of fat cells. When appended, unsaturated fats put away in these cells are discharged into course, to eventually meet their destiny of being oxidized, or "copied."

This procedure of discharging unsaturated fats into the blood is called lipolysis and studies show that intermittent fasting is particularly proficient at actuating it.

Together, this expansion in glucagon and lipolysis is an ideal blend for expanding the amount of weight that is lost specifically from fat tissue.

How Intermittent Fasting Affects Your Hormones

Body fat is the body's way for setting aside energy in the form of calories.

The moment we do not eat anything, the body changes a few things to make the put-away energy more easily available.

This has to do with changes in nervous system action, just as a significant change in a few essential hormones.

Here is a part of the things that change in your digestion when you fast:

- **Insulin**: Insulin increments when we eat. when we fast, insulin diminishes drastically. Lower levels of insulin encourage fat consumption.

- **Human Growth Hormone (HGH)**: Levels of growth hormone may increase during a fast, expanding as much as 5 fold. The growth hormone is a hormone that can help fat loss and muscle gain, in addition to other things.

- **Norepinephrine (noradrenaline)**: The nervous system sends norepinephrine to the fat cells, making them separate body fat into free unsaturated fats that can be used for energy.

Strikingly, in spite of what the 5-6 a day generally recommended meals could make you think, intermittent fasting may really build fat consumption.

Fasting for around 48 hours helps digestion by 3.6-14%. In any case, fasting periods that are longer than this can negatively affect digestion.

Intermittent fasting prompts a few changes in the body that make fat consuming simpler. This includes diminished insulin, expanded growth hormone, improved epinephrine flagging.

Intermittent Fasting Helps Keep Muscle When Dieting

One of the most terrible symptoms of dieting is that the body will, in general, consume muscle just as fat.

Surprisingly enough, there are a few studies demonstrating that intermittent fasting might be useful for keeping muscle while losing body fat.

In one survey study, intermittent calorie limitation caused a similar amount of weight loss as continuous one, yet with a very less noticeable decrease in bulk.

In the continuous calorie limitation, the study considers, 25% of the weight loss was bulk, contrasted with just 10% in the intermittent calorie limitation.

Generally speaking, it seems that there is some proof that intermittent fasting can help you with clutching more bulk when dieting, in contrast to continuous calorie limitation.

Intermittent Fasting Makes Healthy Eating Easier

One of the fundamental benefits of intermittent fasting I especially love is its effortlessness.

I, for one, regularly do the 16/8, where I just eat during a specific "eating window" every day.

Rather than eating three to five meals a day, I eat just two, which makes it significantly simpler to keep up my healthy way of life.

The best "diet" for you to hold on to is the one you can adhere to long term. If intermittent fasting makes it simpler for you to adhere to a healthy diet, then it has clear long term benefits not only for weight but for general health too.

One of the main benefits of intermittent fasting is that it makes healthy eating less complex. This may make it simpler to adhere to a healthy diet over the long term.

Chapter 5 Recap

- Intermittent fasting prompts a few changes in the body that make fat consuming simpler. This includes diminished insulin, expanded growth hormone, improved epinephrine flagging.

- There are studies demonstrating that with intermittent fasting you can avoid losing bulk while losing fat.

- Having a lower number of meals, intermittent fasting helps you to put more care in what you need, even if there are not strict directions about what to eat, chances are that you will naturally end up eating healthier and cleaner

Chapter 6.

Intermittent Fasting and Other Diets

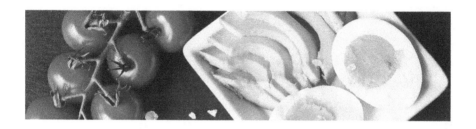

As we now know, intermittent fasting is not exactly a diet, meaning it does not prescribe particular foods or exact amounts of macronutrients. This is why you can generally combine any diet you may be following with intermittent fasting.

Of course, if you are following any diet that requires a continuous intake of nutrients you can't fit it in a fasting plan.

But in general, combining your regular diet with intermittent fasting will only mean that you will just keep following your diet, eating what that diet allows and advises you to eat, but you'll just do it during your feeding windows.

Anyway, integration of intermittent fasting with some diets in particular may need some extra information due to their own peculiarities. Let's see them in detail.

Intermittent Fasting and Keto Diet

The ketogenic diet and intermittent fasting share huge numbers of similar health benefits since the two methods can have a similar outcome: a condition of ketosis.

Ketosis has many physical and mental benefits, from weight and fat loss to improved feelings of anxiety, mental capacity, and life span.

In any case, it's critical to remember that in case you adopt a milder strategy to intermittent keto fasting — for instance, eating inside an 8-hour window — you most likely won't enter ketosis (particularly in the event that you eat a high amount of carbs during that window).

Not everyone who attempts intermittent fasting plans enter ketosis. Indeed, if somebody who fasts also eats high-carb foods, there is a very good chance they will never enter ketosis.

Then again, if ketosis is the objective, you can utilize intermittent keto fasting as an instrument to reach it and improve your overall health.

About biohacking, there most likely are not two more famous practices than the ketogenic high-fat diet and intermittent fasting.

The two regimens have health benefits, including improved digestion, weight loss, and far better immune power.

Ketosis is the process of consuming ketone bodies for energy.

On an ordinary diet, your body consumes glucose as its essential fuel source. Glucose excess is stored as glycogen. At the point when your body is denied glucose (because of exercise, intermittent fasting, or a ketogenic diet), it will go to glycogen for energy. After glycogen is exhausted, will your body begin consuming fat?

A ketogenic diet, which is also called a low-carb, high-fat diet, activates a metabolic move that permits your body to separate fat into ketone bodies in the liver for energy. There are three fundamental ketone bodies found in your blood, pee, and breath:

- **Acetoacetate**: The primary ketone to be made. It can either be changed over into beta-hydroxybutyrate or transformed into CH_32CO (acetone).

- **Acetone**: Created rapidly from the breakdown of acetoacetate. It is the most unpredictable ketone and is frequently perceptible in the breath when somebody initially goes into ketosis.

- **Beta-hydroxybutyrate (BHB)**: This ketone is utilized for energy and the richest in your blood once you are completely in ketosis. It's additionally the type found in exogenous ketones and it's what ketogenic blood tests measure.

Intermittent Fasting and Its Relation to Ketosis

Intermittent fasting comprises eating just inside a particular timeframe and not eating for the rest of the hours of the day. Each person, consciously or not, fast overnight from supper to breakfast.

The benefits of fasting have been utilized for a huge number of years in Ayurveda and Traditional Chinese Medicine as an approach to help reset your digestion and help your gastrointestinal framework subsequent to overeating.

As we now know, there are many different ways to deal with intermittent fasting, with different times: (16-20 hours fasting, alternate-day fasting, 24-hour day fasting,and the other we talked about).

Intermittent fasting can put you in a condition of ketosis faster since your cells will rapidly expand your glycogen stores, and afterward begin utilizing your stored fat for fuel. This prompts an acceleration of the fat-consuming procedure and a ketone levels expansion.

Ketosis and Intermittent Fasting: The Physical Benefits

Both ketogenic diet and the intermittent fasting can be excellent tools for:

- Healthy weight loss

- Fat loss without muscle loss

- Balancing cholesterol levels

- Improving insulin effectiveness

- Keeping glucose levels stable

Ketogenic Diet for Weight Loss, Fat Loss, and Better Cholesterol Levels.

The keto diet radically diminishes your carb intake, compelling your body to consume fat as opposed to glucose. This makes it a successful system for weight loss, yet in addition to the control of diabetes, insulin resistance, and even heart infection.

People who followed a low-carb keto meal plan had loss in body weight, body fat rate, and fat mass, losing an average of 7.6 pounds and 2.6% body fat while keeping up fit bulk.

Watching the long-term effects of a keto diet in overweight people has been found that their weight and body mass diminished drastically over the course of two years. The people who radically diminished their sugar intake saw a critical decline in LDL (bad) cholesterol and triglycerides, and improved insulin effectiveness.

They have compared a ketogenic diet with eating fewer calories in overweight young and adult people. The outcomes indicated kids following the keto diet lost more body weight, fat mass, and waistline. They likewise demonstrated a drop in the insulin levels, the biomarker of type 2 diabetes.

Intermittent Fasting for Fat Loss and Muscle Mass Maintenance

Intermittent fasting can be an effective weight loss instrument, some of the time being significantly more helpful than just limiting your calorie intake.

In one study, intermittent fasting was demonstrated to be as effective as constant calorie limitation in fighting obesity. In studies made by the NIH, weight loss was observed in over 84% of the members, regardless of which fasting plan they picked.

Like ketosis, intermittent fasting can favour fat loss while keeping up fit bulk. In one study, scientists inferred that people who fasted would have better weight loss results (while safeguarding muscle) than the people who followed a low-calorie diet, despite the fact that the all-out caloric intake was equivalent.

Ketosis and Intermittent Fasting: Mental Benefits

Besides their physiological benefits, both intermittent fasting and ketosis give many mental benefits. Both have been experimentally shown to:

- Boost memory

- Improve mental clarity and focus

- Prevent neurological illness including Alzheimer's disease and epilepsy

The effects of Intermittent Fasting on Stress Levels and Cognitive Function

Fasting has been shown to improve memory, decrease oxidative pressure, and help learning abilities.

Researchers accept that intermittent fasting works by forcing cells to perform better. Since your cells are under a slight stress while fasting, the best cells adjust to this stressor by improving their own capacity to adapt, while the most vulnerable cells die. This procedure is called autophagy.

This is like the stress your body experiences when you go to the gym. exercising is a type of stress your body goes through to improve and be more solid, as long as you rest enough after your exercises. This also applies to intermittent fasting, and as long as you keep on shifting back and forth between ordinary dietary patterns and fasting, you can keep on benefiting.

All this implies that keto and intermittent fasting blend is groundbreaking and can help improve your intellectual capacity, because of the defensive and stimulating effects of ketones just as the gentle cell stress brought on by fasting.

Keto and Intermittent Fasting Diet Plan

Possibly you are contemplating trying the keto diet or exploring different ways regarding fasting. Maybe you are now doing both. In any case, here's an example of a day by day and week by week plan of what a plan may look like for somebody on a keto diet, which is also including some alternate day fasting and 16:8 restricted feeding into their routine.

Sunday

6:00 am: Water as well as dark espresso (no, espresso won't break the fast)

9: 00 am: more water or dark espresso.

12:00pm: TRF (time restricted feeding) stops. Have a keto meal: possibly a serving of mixed greens with the flame-broiled chicken breast with olive oil and feta cheese, avocado, and some hard-boiled eggs or bacon slices.

3:00 pm: Snack with some nuts or have some nut butter, and possibly espresso with some MCT oil or coconut oil.

6:00 pm: 8 - 12oz of a greasy cut of meat (ribeye steak or greasy fish) and vegetables, like Brussels sprouts cooked in the spread.

8:00 pm: Small nibble of nuts, blueberries, and a bit of dark chocolate for dessert. This is the last meal of the day.

Monday

It's eating window as yesterday: 12 - 8 pm. On the pattern of Sunday's meal plan.

Tuesday

Fasting day. No calorie intake today.

Wednesday

Eating time 12 - 8 pm. You may be hungrier today since you fasted yesterday, particularly if you did an early morning exercise today.

Thursday

Fasting day.

Friday

Eating time 12 - 8 pm. Workout in the first part of the day or, in the event that you need to do an intense session, do it between lunch and supper.

Saturday

Fast day

Keep in mind; this is just a single model out of an about a boundless number of possibilities! Switch this up to accommodate your way of life; use it as a start to plan your own fasting routine. And in particular, note that this is kind of an advanced plan combining fasting and keto diet, not something you want to start with if you are moving your first steps into intermittent fasting. Remember that you are here to enjoy, not to suffer.

Health Benefits of Keto and Intermittent Fasting

Concentrating on the health benefits of the keto diet and fasting will help you stay focused and keep going on. These benefits can include:

- Decreased levels of insulin

- Reduction of inflammation

- Weight loss

- Heart health

- Lower cholesterol levels and blood pressure

- Autophagy

- Increased energy

- Increased clarity

Keto and Intermittent Fasting Meal Plan Example

Notwithstanding motivation, following the guidelines with respect to what you can eat is a large part of the struggle when you try to do keto and intermittent fasting. An example meal plan follows to make it somewhat simpler. Look at these basic plans.

The following example plan will follow the ketogenic diet alongside 16/8 intermittent fasting. It will be ideal if you note that fasting will happen from 8 pm until noon the next day.

Monday – A glass of water and espresso before Noon. Lunch is a fishplate with mixed greens (canned fish, celery, mayo, avocado cut) and a side serving of mixed greens with farm salad dressing. A snack is a bunch of nuts and cheddar.

Supper is a breadless cheeseburger with spinach, avocado, and mushrooms and a side of zoodles (zucchini noodles).

Tuesday – Start the day with a big glass of water and espresso if you want. Snacks will be made of celery and nut spread. Supper this evening is barbecued sirloin steak basted with mushrooms, simmered broccoli, and cauliflower velouté.

Wednesday – Water and espresso (did you see that coming?). Breakfast for lunch, fried eggs, avocado, and bacon are on the menu. As a snack is a hardboiled egg and a few cucumbers. Supper is salmon cooked with lemon and dill, asparagus, and mixed berries for dessert.

Thursday – Wake up to water and espresso. Lunch is a barbecued chicken plate of mixed greens with hard boiled eggs, avocado, and sunflower seeds. The snack is a serving of olives, pickles, and cheddar. Supper would be cabbage and frankfurter with broccoli, serving of mixed greens as a side (broccoli, mayo, bacon, almonds).

Friday –Morning: water and espresso. Lunch is a sub in a tub (julienne lettuce, tomato, pickles, olives, cheddar, ham, salami, dressed with olive oil and red wine vinegar). Celery sticks with cream cheddar can be added for a touch of crunch. A snack of beef jerky and cheddar. Supper is chicken wings and a side plate of mixed greens with farm salad dressing.

Saturday – Water and espresso before Noon. Lunch is eggroll in a bowl – julienne cabbage, ground pork, and coconut amines (substitutes soy sauce) with a side of kale chips. The bite is nuts and pepperoni. Pizza is for supper, with a cauliflower dough, obviously, alongside a major bowl of broccoli or a side plate of mixed greens.

Sunday – The usual water and espresso. Lunch is a taco serving of mixed greens. Snack comprises veggies and vinaigrette, and supper is a pot soup with green beans and cauliflower cream.

Even if I did not include it, you can also have some dessert after your meal. Some great choices are mixed berries, dark chocolate, or cottage cheese blended in with strawberries. In case you are searching for some keto friendly sweet plans, these may be the ones.

The above menu is only an example of what you can eat. When you become more experienced with the diet and fasting, largely, you will have the option to think of creative recipes to add to your meals. Keeping meals simple helps keep you on target and keep you from getting bored with your food and going to unhealthy choices.

Despite the fact that you can surely nibble during the 8-hour eating window, it is a smart thought to reduce the snacks as you get more accustomed to the keto diet and intermittent fasting. Each time you eat; insulin is discharged, which turns off fat copying for 2-3 hours. In this way, refraining from nibbling will help you in your weight-loss objectives also. Now let's see how we can avoid some common mistakes.

Most Common Mistakes

In case you have been fasting and following the keto diet for a couple of weeks, however not getting in shape – what is the problem? It tends to be so disappointing and makes you need to surrender when you do not get results immediately, yet, there might be a few reasons you are not losing weight.

1. Still too much Carbs

This is presumably the number one suspect for those new to keto and intermittent fasting. Despite the fact that you are eating low carb veggies, there might be sugar alcohols that are causing your weight loss to slow down. Are you actually eating sugar-free products? If this is true, they most likely contain sorbitol, xylitol, or some other sugar alcohol, and you might be eating a lot of them without realizing the effect it is having on you. Many sweeteners can cause raised insulin levels, which slows down your weight loss.

Avoid ready to use dressings and sauces unless you are not sure of their ingredients, as they commonly contain a great deal of hidden carbs.

Pick keto friendly ones rather, for example, those made by Primal Kitchen. Or even better, make your own keto sauces. Home made mayonnaise, for example, is ideal for dressing mixed greens plates. Finding the hidden responsible for slowing down your progress will push you to get back on your way.

2. You Are Not in Ketosis

While you are following the diet on those hard first weeks, you know you are in ketosis; however, that is not always the situation. Keto diet and intermittent fasting beginners are particularly vulnerable to this. Most importantly, you just might be recording and figuring your intake inaccurately. It would be ideal to check, and that should be possible through urine test strips that you can purchase anywhere, from drugstores to the web. For the best precision, get a decent blood ketone screen or ketone breath analyzer.

3. You Are Eating Too Much

Just because you are controlling your carb intake does not mean you can go wild with other foods intake. Eating a larger number of calories than you consume will, in any case, make you put on weight, keto or not. You also should know that the fats you are eating have more calories, so you may need to review the total amount you are having. Likewise, remember that as you get thinner, the amount of calories your body needs will diminish. It is judicious to monitor these information and reevaluate your checks every ten pounds you lose. I strongly suggest utilizing a food tracker, for example, Carb Manager to monitor your food intake.

4. An Excessive Amount of Protein

Here once more, you may need to recalculate your protein needs. An excessive amount of protein can cause gluconeogenesis, a process that changes over protein into sugar. Likewise, you might need to avoid fluid protein, for example, shakes or beverages, as they may change over to sugar faster.

5. Not Fasting Long Enough

In the event that a 16:8 fast is not delivering weight loss, go for a more extended or more constrictive fast, for example, the alternate day fasting. You can begin by doing it once per week and climb your way up to three times each week.

The alternate day fasting is most likely the best fasting type for weight loss. By integrating it with the keto diet, you will experience substantially less appetite accordingly, making it significantly more economical too.

6. Too Much Fasting.

If fasting over 16 hours, you should not fast for consecutive days. Doing as such, over time, can wreck your digestion. You have to enjoy a break from fasting each third week for a time of the multi-week. This helps with resetting your digestion so you can keep profiting by your fasts.

Clearly, in case you are new to keto and intermittent fasting, this will not be an issue for some time. The important thing to keep in mind is that an excess of fasting will, in the end, bring down your digestion. In this way, to avoid weight loss flattening on keto and intermittent fasting, do not fast consecutive days and do not fast for a too large number of weeks straight.

By avoiding the above mistakes, a flattening on keto and intermittent fasting can be forestalled.

Moreover, probably the greatest secret to any fruitful lifestyle is arranging. This is true for Keto and intermittent fasting the same. Finding the occasions that are ideal for you to fast is basic for seeing progress. Planning meals and snacks and sticking to that plan are the basics. Most importantly, you have to know the essentials of the ketogenic diet and how intermittent fasting functions to discover the achievement you look for.

Tips for Success

Most importantly, the way you need to try the keto and intermittent fasting lifestyle is the first step to develop. It is clear that you need to shed pounds and improve your health. It may not always be simple, yet here are a couple of tips to help you follow your path.

1. Track Your Food

There are many apps for you to track the amount of calories, carbs, and truly, whatever else you need to follow. Knowing how much and what you are putting into your body can have a significant effect either on progress and disappointment. Ensure the application is specifically designed for the keto diet.

2. Find a Community

Clearly, changing your way of life can be hard. Not all your loved ones may comprehend your new diet or what you are experiencing. It is imperative to have somewhere you can go and talk and analyze high points and low points or make questions. In case you do not have a companion or mate that is doing the same diet with you then, do not fear, many online networks can help spur and bolster you in your times of hardship.

3. Continue Onward

The moment you first begin with the keto diet and fasting, you may see the weight fall off rapidly, yet then start to slow down. This is the point at which many people choose it is not working for them and quit. You have to remember: it took some time to put that weight on, it will take some to lose it. It is a process, and you will have to stick to it to see the outcomes you want. Regardless of whether you have tumbled off the wagon, you have to dust yourself off and get right back on.

Intermittent fasting and DASH diet

An abbreviation for Dietary Approaches to Stop Hypertension. The DASH diet is demonstrated not only to lower blood pressure, but for its help with weight loss and decrease your danger of many chronic diseases, as well. Low in sodium yet high in potassium, calcium, and magnesium, fruits, veggies, and low fat dairy are the foundation of the DASH diet. Vegetables, nuts and seeds, whole grains, lean meat, and fish are included too.

As for the keto diet, DASH diet is all about the kind of food you eat. Intermittent fasting is about the way you do it. You can effectively combine the two by following the guidelines I gave you about keto and intermittent fasting.

Plant-Based Intermittent Fasting for Vegans

The vegan fasting variant of intermittent fasting can bring splendid results, in spite of the fact that it could, in any case, be a challenging process even for the most committed of vegans.

The 4 Basic Steps to Get Started with Intermittent Vegan Fasting:

1. **Create a feasible plan**: Take a gander at your life, your work hours, and your propensities. Do you, usually, only have a snack at lunch? Do you skip breakfast frequently? Would you be able to quit food for quite a while, or do you get bad-tempered rapidly?

2. **Adopt it gradually**: there is no compelling reason to immediately "dive into deep water" and make your body feel that out of nowhere it is going to starve to death. If it should work better for you, take a stab at the beginning with a 10-hour or 12-hour eating window before dropping down to the 8-hour window. Likewise, in case you are making the 5:2 method , attempt it as a 6:1 diet at the beginning.

3. **Set an audit date**: Set an end date for your fasting, regardless of whether it is two weeks or 2 months from now. If you have not gotten the outcomes you were

seeking after by, at that point, maybe intermittent fasting is not the correct eating plan for you.

4. **Plan your food**: Okay, the general purpose of fasting is that you should not meal plan excessively. In any case, in case you are eating a crude vegan or plant-based diet, you have to search out nutrients and fiber-filled meals, which will limit your craving and hunger during any fast periods.

Vegans Who Should Try Intermittent Fasting

• Vegans who need to get thinner: vegan weight loss is, in fact, achievable with fasting; making it simpler for you to shed pounds and get the body you want.

• Vegans who need to improve their performance at the gym: studies propose that intermittent fasting supports development hormones by as much as 500%.

• Vegans who need to grow better dietary patterns: some vegans eat unhealthy food absentmindedly. Plant-based intermittent fasting forces you to create healthier dietary patterns.

Vegans Who Should Not Try Intermittent Fasting

Vegans who are pregnant or breastfeeding: If you are a vegan who is pregnant or breastfeeding, try not to explore new ways about diets and fasting methods. Your infant is developing and is depending on you for a consistent intake of nutrients.

Vegans who are diabetic: Although a few sources guarantee that fasting could help with diabetes, it is largely prescribed that diabetics ought not to fast, as the procedure could upset their glucose levels. So if you are diabetic and want to try Intermittent fasting, always consult your doctor, and follow their directions.

Chapter 6 Recap

- Unless you are following a diet that requires a continuous intake of nutrients, you will quite easily be able to fit your current diet in an intermittent fasting plan.

- The ketogenic diet and intermittent fasting share huge numbers of similar health benefits since the two methods can have a similar outcome: a condition of ketosis.

- DASH diet is all about the kind of food you eat, intermittent fasting is about the how and when. You can effectively combine the two diets.

- You can integrate your vegan diet with intermittent fasting, just be aware, even more than you usually are, of the balance of the nutrients you take in.

Chapter 7.

The Importance of Lifestyle

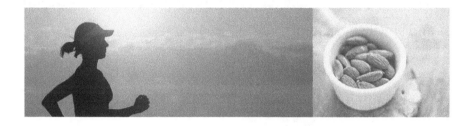

Once you get started with intermittent fasting you will soon notice a natural tendency towards a more generally healthy lifestyle. This is a quite common virtuous circle: you start with a single healthy choice, this makes you feel better, feeling better gives you the energy to go on with more healthy choices, in a snowball effect of wellness.

You will naturally know and feel what healthy changes you'll need to put into your life, and this will probably not only concern body's health, but mind and spirit too. For instance, once I kept experiencing an increase in clarity, I naturally felt the desire to read more books and scheduled a daily "me-time" of 45 minutes, just me and my book, door closed and phone off.

So, now we are going to look at some aspects you should consider as a general lifestyle background for your intermittent fasting path, still, this is just some advice, please listen to yourself and be ready to embrace your body, mind and spirit suggestions.

Moderate, if you don't want to get rid of, alcohol

Intermittent fasting has shown to diminish inflammation in your body.

In any case, alcohol may aggravate inflammation, limiting the benefits of this diet.

Chronic inflammation may advance different diseases, for example, heart disease, type 2 diabetes, and certain malignancies.

Research shows that inflammation from excessive drinking may prompt intestinal disorder, bacterial overgrowth, and anomalies in intestinal microorganisms.

High alcohol intake can likewise strain your liver, diminishing its capacity to sift through possibly damaging elements.

Together, these consequences for your intestine and liver may advance inflammation all through your body, which over time can cause organ harm.

Over the top alcohol intake can cause far-reaching inflammation in your body, slowing if not stopping the effects of intermittent fasting and conceivably prompting infections.

Also, consider that drinking alcohol can break your fast

During a fast, you should avoid all foods and drinks for a certain amount of time.

In particular, intermittent fasting is intended to advance hormonal and physical changes —, for example, fat consuming and cell repair— that may benefit your health.

As alcohol contains calories, any amount of it during a fasting period will break your fast. Apart from that, it is perfectly acceptable to drink in moderation during your eating periods.

During fasting periods, your body starts cell repair processes like autophagy, in which old, harmed proteins are expelled from cells to produce more effective, healthier cells.

This process may diminish your danger of malignancy, distances the issues of ageing effects, and at any rate, somewhat clarifies why calorie limitation has been shown to expand life expectancy.

Ongoing animal studies showing that constant alcohol intake may hinder autophagy in the liver and fat tissue.

Picking better alcohol choices

As alcohol breaks your fast whenever expended during a fasting period, it is recommended to just drinking during your planned eating periods. You should likewise hold your intake under tight restraints. Moderate alcohol consumption is characterized as close to one drink a day for women and close to two a day for men.

While intermittent fasting does not have exacting standards for food and drink intake, some alcohol habits are healthier than others are and more averse to hinder your dietary routine.

To restrict your sugar and calorie intake, avoid cocktails and prefer wines. During intermittent fasting, it is ideal to drink alcohol moderately and only during your eating windows.

The Unhindered Eating Trap

Anyone who has ever changed their diet to get a health benefit or a healthy weight realizes that you begin to desire foods that you are recommended not to eat. Truth be told, a study published in 2017 affirmed that an increased drive to eat is a key factor during a weight loss journey.

Nevertheless, this test is explicitly restricted on an intermittent fasting plan. Food limitation just happens during certain restricted hours, and on the non-fasting hours or days of the plan, you can, for the most part, eat anything you desire.

Obviously, keeping on with unhealthy foods may not be the healthiest way to pick up benefits from intermittent fasting; however, removing them during specific days restricts your overall intake and may in the end give benefits anyway.

Don't stop working out

Or start doing it if you didn't.

You don't need to be an athlete, but you can't afford a sedentary lifestyle. Some people may think that since they are fasting they should save energy and rest a lot. Well, that's not exactly like this. You should exercise as much as you can (that could be a little, for you, but still), just taking some care.

You should choose whether you would want to work out while fasting or after having eaten. On the chance that you stick to the early afternoon to 8 P.M. eating plan, this mainly comes down to whether you usually work out in the first part of the day or in the evening. Remember that you can change your timetable to your necessities. If you want to work out toward the beginning of the day after eating, you can change your fasting and eating periods to do it.

Training During Fasting

Training in a fasted state requires a few supplements to keep your body in an anabolic state. The body utilizes amino acids for energy if you are training without a pre-exercise meal. Your supplements for fast ought to include glutamine and branched-chain amino acid (BCAA) supplement.

Following the early afternoon to 8 P.M. feeding plan, you fast from 8 P.M. until around noon. So, take your glutamine and BCAA enhancements, and then, do your workout. Depending on how long your workout will last, this will set your post-exercise meal around early afternoon.

What number of meals you decide to have during your starting period is up to you, however, remember that eating less as often as possible can hold your yearning within proper limits and support your body's capacity to build muscle.

Training During Feeding Period

On the chance that you like to work out after eating, you can plan your exercise to fall in the afternoon (early around 1 pm, or toward the evening, around 5 pm). If your workout session is for the most part in the late afternoon, have your pre-training meal around the early afternoon, work out, and afterwards have your other meals.

For an evening session, have your first meal around early afternoon and your pre-exercise meal around 4 P.M. If you may want to have a post-training meal one hour after working out, you can do that, too.

Adjusting Your Calorie Intake

The main principles about intermittent fasting include a few directions of when and how to get your calories and macronutrients.

If you will train while fasting, the calorie check of your BCAA supplement should be calculated toward your complete calories of the day, even though it does not end your fasting period. People on intermittent fasting plans normally distribute fifty calories for their fasting period to take into account things like supplements or refreshments. This implies you can, in any case, take cream and sugar in your espresso or tea, regardless of whether or not it is during your fasting period.

In case you eat a pre-training meal, it is preferable to keep it light. Your meal should include a protein source like poultry or fish and some carbs, for a total amount of 400-500 calories. This will give you the protein and complex starches that are often suggested for pre-exercise meals. If you do eat a pre-exercise meal, the BCAA supplements prescribed for fasting exercises are most likely redundant, but you might need to take them in any case, since having an overflow of BCAAs may now be helpful anyway.

Your post-training meal is the best time to take a large portion of your sugars and calories. About a big part of your total calories for the day ought to be eaten during your post-training meal.

Conclusion

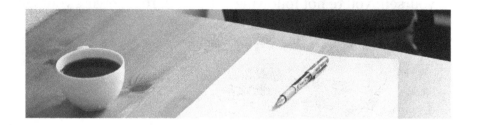

Well, this is it I guess.

I hope you enjoyed reading this book at least as much as I enjoyed writing it. But even more, I hope that this reading may have been a push for you to take action, because you know, you won't get fitter, healthier or thinner just by reading a book.

Again, I want to stress my main point about this diet: of course you have now some technical information, some ideas, some hints about a better lifestyle related to intermittent fasting. And this is great. Though, the main thing about this, or any other, diet, is not how it technically works. It is that you should enjoy it. You should visualize your goal and then love the journey, whatever the reasons behind your decision of taking this path they all are the same reason: you love yourself, and you want to act like it.

So that's what you have to do, loving yourself, taking care of yourself: you're not following a diet, you're following yourself.

If you have liked this book I would love to know. A review on amazon would be appreciated, of course. But even more I would love to hear from you. What you did like about the book, what I could have done better, any kind of congratulation or criticism would be really appreciated. so please feel free to write to me at zhellenberry@gmail.com. I'd be happy to read from you and I always try to reply to every message.

CPSIA information can be obtained
at www.ICGtesting.com
Printed in the USA
BVHW090932141220
595665BV00010B/416

9 781801 118569